HOMEM

HAND SANITIZER

The ultimate guide to making 15 different hand sanitizers at home by easy and fast recipes using simple ingredients.

Protect yourself from germ, bacterial and infections

Nicholas Mitchell

Table of Contents

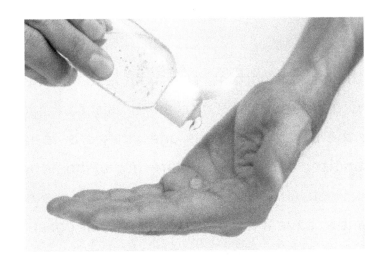

Introduction

One of the most important recommendation by the World Health Organization (WHO) to avoid viral contagion and to stop the spread of germs and viruses is to use the hand sanitizer gel. When we are not at home and we need to wash our hands without soap and water, it is important to have a hand sanitizer gel that doesn't need rinsing and that allows you to sanitize your hands immediately after touching products, materials and surfaces. Unfortunately, hand sanitizers stocks run out and these products are difficult to find in pharmacies, supermarkets and all shops, so it is inevitable to use DIY products. Millions of people who need to go out for work or emergencies are in crisis due to the shortage of pocket sanitizers, but fortunately creating a DIY hand sanitizer gel is very simple, as are protective masks. However, it is important to be careful not to spoil everything, you must be sure that the tools used for the mixtures are properly disinfected otherwise you could increase the risk to contaminate everything. In this guide we will see 10 different recipes to prepare an alcohol-based hand sanitizer at home and 5 recipes to prepare Alcohol-Free sanitizers (which are not disinfectants).

Before to start, we remember some basic rules that must be followed to protect yourself and the people around you:

What to do

- Wash your hands regularly for 40-60 seconds with soap and water or an alcohol-based product

- When coughing or sneezing, cover your nose and mouth with a disposable handkerchief or with the hollow of elbow

- Avoid close contact with people who are not well (keep one meter away)

- If you do not feel well, stay at home and isolate yourself from other family members

What not to do

- Touching eyes, nose and mouth with unclean hands

How to Wash Your Hands

In emergency situations it is very important to wash your hands by following rules and being careful. Washing your hands is not something to be underestimated for the safety of everyone. In most cases (arrival at the office, back home, restaurant) we can wash our hands: hand washing, with a certain frequency and in the correct way, using a normal soap, is still considered the most effective way to prevent infections. Liquid soap is strongly recommended because it is not exposed to air and therefore does not allow germs to proliferate, as can happen on the surface of the solid soap.

World Health Organization (WHO) recommends 10 simple steps to wash your hands using just soap and water to avoid any risks of contamination. The following are the steps to perform:

1. Wet your hands with clean, running water

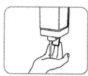

2. Apply enough soap to cover the entire surface of the hands

3. Rub your palms together

4. Right palm over the left back and vice versa interlacing the fingers together

5. Palm against palm by interlacing the fingers

6. Back of the fingers against the palm keeping the fingers tight between the

 7. Rub your left thumb into your right palm and vice versa

 8.Rotational rubbing of the right hand fingers on left hand palm and vice versa

 9.Rinse your hands with water

 10.Use the towel to turn off the tap

After you dry them, your hands will be safe!

Remember to wash your wrists too, especially if you are wearing a watch where viruses and bacteria could nest. The procedure should take between 40 and 60 seconds, you could sing the famous song "Happy birthday" twice to make sure you have washed your hands for the minimum time needed (with this trick you will be sure you have used about 40 seconds). Try now!

Different types of hand sanitizer

A sanitizing product can be useful in situations where we cannot wash our hands with soap and water. However, there are some differences among all products that we find on the market.

Some of them can be very effective, especially in particular situations. But which ones are worth buying? Before explaining the main categories, let's say it again: when you can, wash your hands. In fact, water and a normal soap remain the first choice. If you touch the handle of a public bathroom, you are sure to find a sink with soap nearby, such as when you come back home or to the office, soap and water are always available.

There are different types of hand sanitizers on the market, there are those alcohol-based, those alcohol-free, in gel, spray and foam format. We see below the main features.

Alcohol based

When there is no water you can use sanitizers if they have an alcoholic base. Remember that they must be used on dry hands, otherwise they are ineffective. The presence of alcohol has the purpose of acting directly on the vitality of microbes, killing a good part of them. Attention, however, not all products have the same alcohol concentration and not all formulations (gel, liquid or foam) have the same effectiveness (for example, according to WHO the gel formula is less effective disinfectant). The alcohol on the label can be indicated in different ways (alcohol denat, isopropanol, ethanol, 1-propanol) but as we said its concentration that is important: it is effective only if the alcohol is in a concentration between 60% and 95%. Some of these products are classified as cosmetics (such as common soap) and do not show the percentage of alcohol. Others, on the other hand, are classified as medical-surgical devices, and indicate the amount of alcohol they contain.

As we have seen, products containing 60-95% alcohol are considered effective against bacteria, viruses and fungi. Is not needed the concentration at 95%, because it is not necessarily more effective than a gel with a lower concentration. The WHO, in its indications on the production of alcohol-based gels, suggests a solution based on 80% ethanol or 75% isopropanol. For this reason, all homemade sanitizer done using Vodka or similar are not useful because the alcohol concentration is about 40% in vodka. It is important to consider that alcohol-based sanitizers help to quickly reduce the number of germs on the hands in some situations, but not to eliminate them all. They are also not suitable for cleaning dirty hands or removing harmful chemicals from hands. In these cases, wash your hands with soap and water. Whether they are "simple" cosmetics or medical-surgical devices, there is not necessarily a need for them, on the contrary: if they contain antimicrobial substances you have to be very careful because the unnecessary and unconditional use could encourage the development of resistance in bacteria against these products.

Moreover, alcohol-based products have the disadvantage of drying the skin very much, so continued use can have negative effects on the skin. Similarly, the excessive hand washing in the long term may also cause undesired effects, such as excessive dryness and irritation, although it is needed for some professions.

Alcohol free

Alcohol-free sanitizing gels use other agents such as benzalkonium chloride or triclosan, but a number of considerations need to be made. While effective in fighting bacteria, after a prolonged period of use, bacteria can develop resistance to some of the agents used in alcohol-free gels, (which is not the case with alcohol). It is also necessary to know that some of the ingredients of alcohol-free gels are environmentally harmful and, when combined with other agents, can even become toxic. Finally, in contrast to alcohol-based gels, alcohol-free gels are more susceptible to contamination, which can impair their effectiveness.

Gel VS Spray

The gel format is the most popular, especially because it can be used without water. These types of gel sanitizers should be rubbed in your hands for at least 1 minute. They are also used in sprays format on the hands and on the palms, to be rubbed for 1 minute, repeated for another minute and then left to dry. The choice is often personal, the spray version could be a good choice, but the dispenser may not work properly or clog. The gel version instead has a simple container with a cap that can be easily found at home. The gel finally dries and absorbs much faster than spray solutions being liquid, but the latter are considered more effective.

How to use hand sanitizer

When the hands are not dirty or visibly stained, the sanitizing gel could be a valid alternative, according to the health authorities, since it is believed to kill 99.9% of the bacteria present on the hands in just 30 seconds. For it to work, however, it is necessary to apply it correctly, as is also often shown by signs in hospitals:

1. Apply a little bit of product on the hand palm;
2. Place the two palms against each other and massage to distribute the product;
3. Braid the hands, rubbing well between the fingers;
4. Continue by placing the backs of the two hands against each other and continue rubbing.

For effective cleaning, attention must be paid to nooks, crannies and exposed surface areas that are often not cleaned carefully, such as the areas around the nails, between the fingers, thumb area and wrist. In total the cleaning process should take at least 30 seconds and then let your hands dry (but in any case the gel absorbs very quickly). It is also advisable to remove any rings or bracelets when washing your hands. The sanitizing gel does not require rinsing, on the contrary, washing your hands after applying the gel cancels its effectiveness. Doctors recommend using the sanitizer gel in several situations, including:

- **before:** preparing a meal, eating, treating a wound or taking medicine, touching a sick or injured person, putting on or taking off contact lenses;

- **after:** preparing a meal, using the toilet, changing a diaper, touching an animal, an animal's toy and leash, blowing your nose, coughing or sneezing, touching an injured or sick person, taking out the garbage or touching dirty objects such as shoes, travelling on public transport.

Homemade hand sanitizer

There are different procedures to prepare a hand sanitizing gel; we will see some recipes based on alcohol, others without alcohol, fragrant and natural. Most of the recipes use some basic components: alcohol, aloe vera, glycerin and essential oils such as Tea Tree oil. It is clear that much will depend on what is available at home. However, it could be a good way to spend your time especially if you are bored at home and to save money considering that unfortunately the prices of sanitizer gel on market are increasing considerably. Preparing a DIY gel could be one of the things to do during your stay at home.

The first homemade hand sanitizer that you can prepare is the one that the WHO (World Health Organization) suggests and you can surely make it with what you already have in the pantry or under the sink and it will be effective in emergency situations. Other recipes using different ingredients with different characteristics and flavors will also be illustrated. There are some recipes a bit more complex, in this case you will need to buy some products if you do not already have them available at home. Many of these items, especially when there is an emergency, quickly run out and it is easier to find them in some smaller store, but be careful, since it is more important to stay at home, go out only if it is strictly necessary.

Well, if you are ready, below are the ingredients used and where you can find them, then you can start preparing your first homemade sanitizer!

Where to find the required ingredients

Before presenting the recipes, it is very useful to know where to find the main ingredients if you do not already have them at home:

- Ethanol 96% - Supermarket
- Glycerin (100% vegetable) - E-cigarettes shops, Web shop
- Distilled water (or boiled water) - Supermarket, pharmacy
- Hydrogen peroxide - Supermarket, pharmacy
- Aloe vera gel - Pharmacy, herbalist shop, big supermarket or check here:
  https://www.walgreens.com/q/aloe+vera+gel
  https://www.walmart.com/c/kp/aloe-vera-gel
  https://www.globosurfer.com/best-aloe-vera-gel
- Aloe vera plant - Florist, big supermarket
- Essential oils (Tea Tree, eucalyptus, lavender, cloves, cinnamon, lemon, oregano, thyme, rosemary) - Pharmacy, herbalist shop, big supermarket or check here:
  https://www.enfleurage.com/categories/essential-oils/

https://www.health.com/beauty/tea-tree-oil-benefits

- Liquid bicarbonate - Pharmacy, herbalist shop, big supermarket
- Bleach – Supermarket
- Allantoin - Cosmetics shop, or check here: https://www.bulkactives.com/product/product/allantoin.html
- Carbopol ultrez - Cosmetics shop, or check here: https://www.glamourcosmetics.it/gb/carbopol-ultrez-21
- Sodium hydroxide 20% solution - Cosmetics shop, or check here: https://www.flowertalescosmetics.com/en/catalogue/product/sodium-hydroxide-caustic-soda-20-solution
- Carrageenan – Cosmetics shop, Supermarket or check here: https://www.walmart.com/ip/Kappa-Carrageenan-8-Oz/993278334 https://www.specialingredients.it/carrageenan-iota-100g

- Panthenol - Cosmetics shop, or check here: https://www.aromantic.co.uk/products/d-panthenol
- White or apple vinegar – Supermarket
- Witch Hazel - Cosmetics shop, or check here: https://www.iherb.com/c/witch-hazel

Aloe vera and Tea tree oil properties

As many people know, the two most used ingredients for the hand sanitizers are Aloe vera and Tea tree essential oil. Let's see why and their main characteristics.

Aloe vera

Aloe (Aloe barbadensis Miller) is a plant with long, thick dark green leaves with yellow spots, consisting of an outer part containing a bitter latex and an inner part consisting of a gelatinous layer. Native to tropical Africa, it now grows also in the other continents.

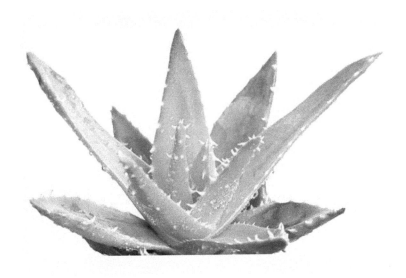

A lot of products containing Aloe gel for external use are very common: as a healing and antibacterial for some dermatological problems, in case of burns, burns, or psoriasis, but also as a simple moisturizer or sunscreen. In addition to the cosmetics sector: fluids, creams, lotions, balms and compresses for the face, lips and body.

If you have an Aloe plant at home, you could easily cut a leaf with a knife and remove the gel. Try to put it on your hands and you will immediately feel a pleasant sensation of softness and hydration.

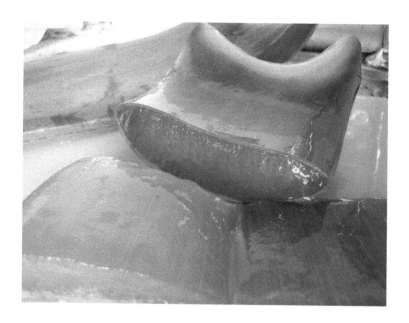

Tea tree oil

Tea tree essential oil is a multifunctional extract obtained from the leaves of Melaleuca alternifolia, a plant widespread in the marshy areas of the Australian east coast. The name of the product, coined in the eighteenth century by the English sailors landed in Australia, often leads to confusion, even if they have nothing in common, with the tea plant (Camellia sinensis) from which are taken the leaves used to produce the black and green tea.

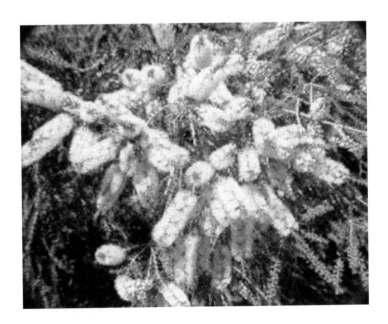

An essential oil is extracted from the leaves, with a very strong smell and intense and unique taste, which has the famous properties attributed to this plant.

Melaleuca essential oil is a powerful antiseptic, antifungal, antibacterial and antiviral, as well as being slightly anesthetic.

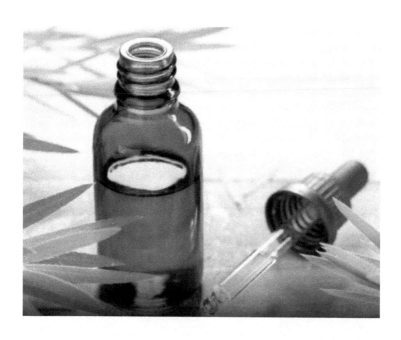

10 Alcohol based recipes

Recipe 1: WHO recommended Homemade hand sanitizer

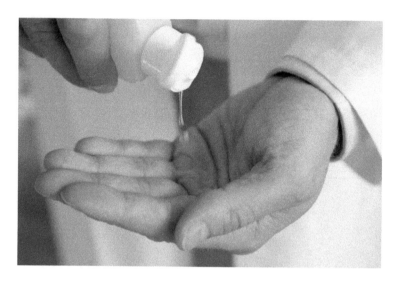

Ingredients for 1 litre:

- Ethanol 96%: 833 ml
- Hydrogen peroxide 3%: 40 ml
- Glycerol 98%: 15 ml
- Distilled water just enough to reach one liter (or water first boiled and then cooled, be careful not to use hot water to avoid toxic inhalations)

Instructions:

The water used must be distilled or boiled and then cooled. To prepare the alcohol-based hand disinfectant we would need a well-cleaned container where the level of one litre is marked. The container can be made of plastic or glass, while the solution can be mixed with plastic, metal or wooden tools. Proceed by pouring 833 ml of alcohol, then with a syringe, take 40 ml of hydrogen peroxide and mix it with the alcohol. Take 15 ml of glycerine and dilute it in the solution. Proceed with patience as the glycerine is very dense. Mix everything well and add the water previously boiled and cooled until it reaches the total volume of one litre. We have thus prepared 1 litre of liquid hand sanitizer that can be used to fill our pocket bottles and those of the people we want.

Recipe 2: Sweet almond Pocket Gel

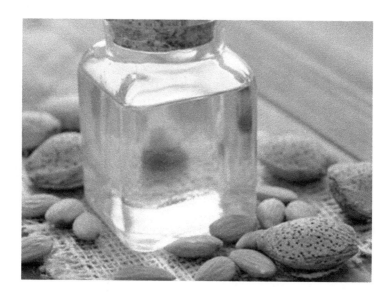

Ingredients for a 75 ml small bottle:

- Ethanol 96%: 6 tablespoons
- Aloe vera gel: 4 tablespoons
- Sweet almond oil: 1 teaspoon
- Tea tree essential oil: 5 drops

Instructions:

Mix all the ingredients together and pour the mixture into a small bottle. It will keep for about a month. Keep in mind that a hand sanitizing gel, to be really effective, should contain at least 60% alcohol.

Recipe 3: Eucalyptus Cheap Gel

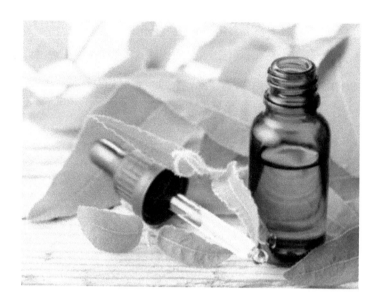

Ingredients:

- Isopropyl alcohol: 150 ml
- Tea tree essential oil: 15 drops
- Eucalyptus essential oil: 30 drops
- Aloe vera gel: 100g – 3.5 oz

Instructions:

Mix the essential oils together and add the alcohol. Finally add the aloe and pour the mix into a corked container and shake well before using it. To increase the disinfectant action of the tea tree and give the product a citrus scent you can add 5 drops of bergamot or lemon essential oil.

Recipe 4: Lavender & Cloves Gel

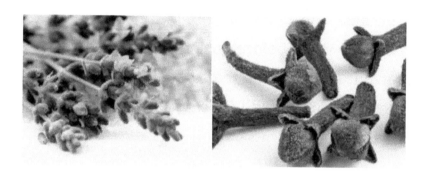

Ingredients:

- Isopropyl alcohol: 150 ml
- Aloe vera gel: 100g – 3.5 oz
- Lavender essential oil: 10 drops
- Clove oil: 10 drops
- Tea tree essential oil: 10 drops

Instructions:

Pour 10 drops of each essential oil and aloe gel into a bowl and mix well. Then add the alcohol, pour the mixture into an old recycling vial and keep it away from light.

Recipe 5: Nick's secret sanitizer gel

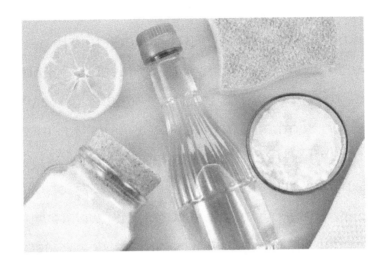

Ingredients:

- Water: 40gr – 1,4oz
- Carrageenan: 2gr – 0.07oz
- Glycerin: 10gr – 0.4oz
- Ethanol 96%: 45gr – 1.6oz
- Tea tree essential oil: 8 drops
- Lavender essential oil: 10 drops
- Lemon essential oil: 10 drops

Instructions:

Put a glass on a precision scale and pour 40gr (1,4oz) of water. Then add 2gr (0.07oz) of carrageenan that is a natural gelling agent used in cosmetics and food. You can find it in online stores that sell cosmetic raw materials as suggested in this guide. Stir with a teaspoon for about 10 minutes to moisturize the carrageenan. Leave the mixture for another 10 minutes and in the meantime weigh the other ingredients, then put 45gr (1,6oz) of alcohol in another glass. Add 10gr (0,40z) of glycerine and the essential oils to the alcohol. Mix well to solubilize the essential oils using a teaspoon. Whisk the water with carrageenan to form a very dense gel using the immersion mixer. Gradually add the alcohol solution by stirring from time to time (do not be in a hurry). Finally, you can add 2 drops of food coloring to personalize your sanitizing gel. Mix well and pour everything into a small container for your bag or a dispenser to keep at home!

Recipe 6: Amuchina spray

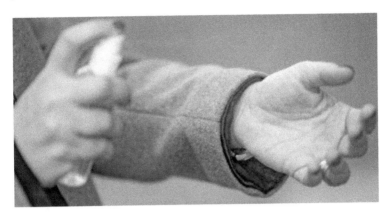

Ingredients:

- Bleach
- Distilled water
- Ethanol 96%: 74gr - 2,6 oz
- Amuchina (done before): 26gr 0,92 oz
- Essential oil as you like

Instructions:

Dilute the bleach (1 part bleach 2 part water) to obtain the low-cost version of the amuchina. Pour the alcohol (74gr-2,6oz) in a glass container and add the low cost amuchina (26gr-0.92oz). Mix and add the essential oil to taste. Pour it all into a spray bottle and your sanitizer is ready

Recipe 7: Carbopol Power

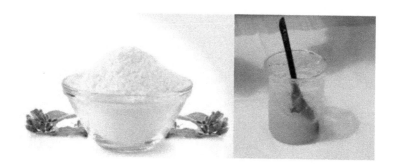

Ingredients:

- Water: 26,20 gr - 92,4oz
- Allantoin: 0,15gr – 0.01oz
- Carbopol ultrez 21: 1,15 gr – 0.04oz
- Glycerine: 1,5gr – 0.05oz
- Glycolic ether of marigold (or other): 1gr – 0.03oz
- Ethanol 96%: 70gr – 2.5oz
- Mint Essential: 6 drops
- Sodium hydroxide: 6-7 drops

Instructions:

Heat the water slightly and add allantoin in a small glass container, mix well and let the water cool. Add the dose of carbopol, usually carbopol needs more water so you need to hydrate it very well especially if carbopol is not new (don't hurry, let it hydrate even half an hour). When carbopol is perfectly hydrated add the glycolic extract and glycerine that is needed to hydrate the hands (it is important because of the doses of alcohol to avoid drying the hands). Mix everything with a teaspoon. Bring to PH 5.5 - 6 by adding 6-7 drops of a soda solution to harden the gel (otherwise it will soften) and mix (it will be hard enough). If you have PH strip cards you can check the value. Now you can start adding 96% alcohol but be careful little by little! (one teaspoon at a time and stir). Don't be in a hurry to add the alcohol to make the gel more liquid...! When the gel is ready add a few drops of mint essential oil and mix. The gel will become softer! Finally add the dye you like and put the gel in a small travel bottle using a syringe.

Recipe 8: Oregano

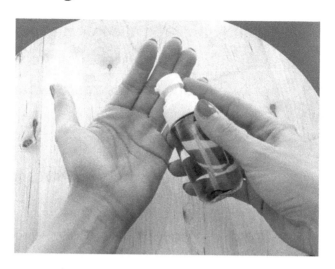

Ingredients:

- Aloe vera gel: 40gr – 1,4oz
- Ethanol 96%: 50gr – 1,8oz
- Oregano essential oil: 6 drops

Instructions:

Mix 40 g of liquid aloe vera gel (about 4 tablespoons) with 50 g of food grade 96° ethyl alcohol (about 6 tablespoons) and 6 drops of Oregano essential oil, a powerful natural antibacterial, one of the best to use. Pour the mixture into a dispenser bottle well cleaned and sanitized. Both ingredients can be purchased in organic shops and herbalist shops or in quality organic online shops. In this recipe we use liquid aloe gel to increase the storage capacity instead of the plant. The essential oil of oregano has the following properties: antiseptic, lipolytic, antifungal, parasiticide, antiviral, antibacterial, tonic.

Recipe 9: Lemon gel

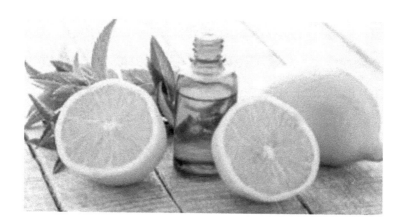

Ingredients:

- Water: 50ml
- Carrageenan: 1,5 tablespoons
- Ethanol 96%: 50ml
- Vegetable Glycerine
- Lemon essential oil: 10ml
- Food coloring: 5 drops

Instructions:

Put the water in a container, add the carrageenan and stir with a teaspoon. Let the carrageenan hydrate well for at least 20 minutes. Put the 96 % alcohol in another container and add the vegetable glycerine, stir well with a teaspoon. Combine the two mixtures and blend everything by adding the alcohol a little at a time. Finally add the lemon essential oil and the food coloring agent. Continue blending to make the gel homogeneous in color. Pour the gel into a plastic travel bottle using a syringe (without needle) or a funnel.

Recipe 10: WHO Homemade hand sanitizer variant

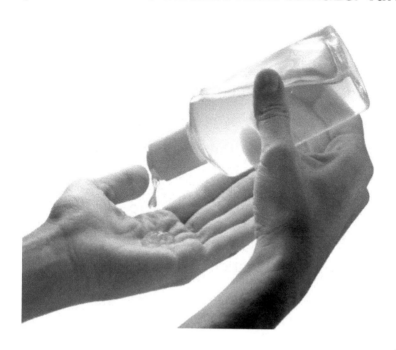

Ingredients for 1 litre:

- Isopropyl alcohol 80%: 888ml
- Hydrogen peroxide 3%: 5 tablespoons
- Glycerine 98%: 2 tablespoon
- Distilled water (or boiled and then cooled): 7 tablespoons
- Essential oil as you prefer

Instructions:

Pour the Isopropyl alcohol into a plastic bottle using a funnel and add hydrogen peroxide. Shake and add 2 tablespoons of glycerine. Finally add 7 tablespoons of distilled water and shake. Remember that alcohol only disinfects if you add the right amount of water. Considering that Isopropyl alcohol is cheaper than food alcohol (Ethanol 96%) but has a bad smell so it is recommended to add a few drops of essential oil as you like.

5 Alcohol free recipes

Following recipes are alcohol free so do not consider them as real disinfectants but as excellent soap and water alternatives when you're away from home.

Recipe 1: Cinnamon & Lemon

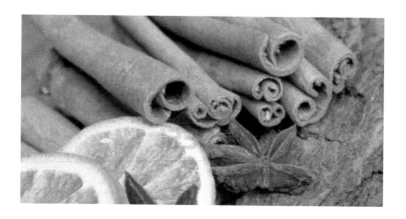

Ingredients:

- Aloe vera: 2 tablespoons
- Cinnamon essential oil: 15 drops
- Lemon essential oil: 12 drops
- Water: 100ml

Instructions:

Get a dispenser vial that previously contained liquid soap and wash it thoroughly. Use aloe vera gel as a base, two tablespoons will be enough.

Add 15 drops of cinnamon essential oil and 12 lemon essential oil. Dilute with 100 ml of water and mix everything together. Shake well before use to mix the oils.

Recipe 2: Thyme and rosemary

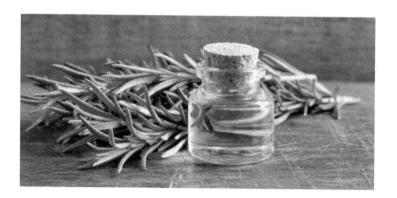

Ingredients:

- Liquid bicarbonate: 20 ml
- Aloe Vera: 30 ml
- Tea tree oil: 5 drops
- Thyme essential oil: 5 drops
- Rosemary essential oil: 5 drops of

Instructions:

Extract the pulp from an aloe vera leaf (if you don't have a real plant, pure aloe vera gel on the market will be fine too). Proceed by inserting the pulp into a mixer to obtain the Aloe Vera gel. Then combine all the ingredients, mix until a homogeneous gel is obtained and pour it into a container with a dispenser.

Recipe 3: Orange and mint

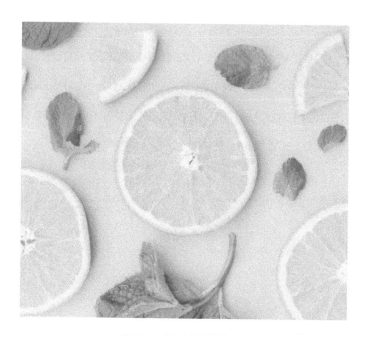

Ingredients:

- Liquid bicarbonate: 20 ml
- Aloe Vera: 30 ml
- Tea tree oil: 5 drops
- Orange essential oil: 5 drops
- Mint essential oil: 5 drops

Instructions:

Choose a large aloe vera leaf and cut it at the base with a sharp knife. Place the leaf on a flat surface and cut the edges and tip. To extract the gel, you can use the knife or a teaspoon. At this point insert the gel into the blender and blend. Now you just have to add all the ingredients, mix them and pour the gel obtained into a container with dispenser that you can use whenever and wherever you want.

Recipe 4: Natural and Fast

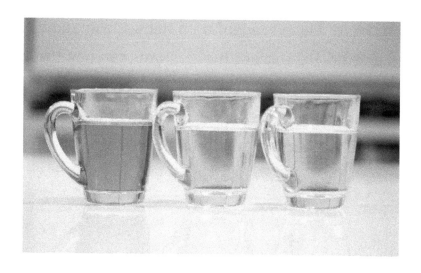

Ingredients:

- White vinegar (or apple vinegar): 49 ml
- Water: 49ml
- Tea tree essential oil: 2ml (40 drops approx.)
- 100 ml spray bottle

Instructions:

Fill a 200ml plastic bottle with all the ingredients, put the cap and shake well to have a good emulsion. You can spray the mixture on your hands when you do not have soap and water available, or after washing your hands as an additional precaution, but always remember to shake the mixture before using it to restore the emulsion.

If you want to increase the disinfectant effect of the vinegar as much as possible, you can prepare another spray bottle of the same size but filled with hydrogen peroxide. Spray the vinegar mixture on your hands first and then the one with hydrogen peroxide.

Recipe 5: Witch hazel

For those who do not want to use alcohol there are, as seen above, other alternatives which, however, as said before, do not have the same effectiveness on an antibacterial level. In addition to apple vinegar, we propose a variant with witch hazel.

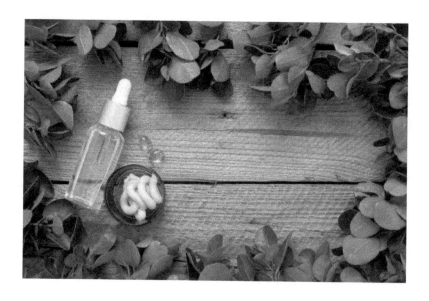

Ingredients:

- Aloe vera gel (preferably without additives): 240ml
- Witch Hazel: 2 teaspoons
- Tea tree oil: 30 drops
- Lavender or mint essential oil: 5 drops of

Instructions:

Mix aloe vera gel, tea tree oil and witch hazel. If you want a thicker gel, add another spoonful of aloe vera. If you want a more liquid product, add another tablespoon of witch hazel. Then add the essential oil, since the smell of tea tree oil is quite intense, do not exaggerate with the added essential oils. Four or five drops should be enough, but if you want to increase the doses, add one drop at a time. Pour the mixture into a container using a funnel. Once filled, close it with the cap until it is ready to use.

If you want to bring your gel during the day, use a small soft plastic bottle that can be squeezed out.

How to make Soap strips

Here you can find an easy way to have always with you the hand soap!

Enjoy!

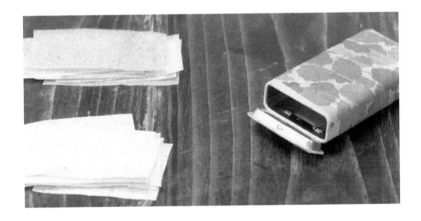

Needed:

- Water-soluble paper
- Eco-friendly liquid dish soap
- Body liquid soap
- Hand liquid soap

Instructions:

Place the water soluble sheet of paper inside a container of the same size and with a brush apply a layer of soap first on both sides. You can do this with 3 sheets using dish soap for the first one, bath foam for the second one and liquid hand soap on the third sheet.

Let the sheets dry in the open air by hanging them with clips on the cables.

When they are dry, cut the sheets into many small rectangles in the size of a candy container. Place the sheets in a candy tin container and carry it with you at all times! Our soap sheets are ready when you're or on the road, just rub them in your hands like a bar of soap under water.

You can buy the water soluble paper here:

https://www.smartsolve.com/shop/water-soluble-paper-it118698

Conclusions

It is important to know that a mixture containing dangerous substances must never be stored in anonymous containers without a label and information about the content and date of preparation.

The do-it-yourself preparations proposed in this guide do not replace those on the market and are not certified. Some ingredients can be dangerous, so be careful when using them and keep them away from heat sources and children.

The WHO (World Health Organization) recommends washing your hands often with soap and water, which remains a good habit to prevent contagion and infection.

Finally, remember that the virus does not have the legs to spread but uses those of man, so stay at home and everything will be fine.

Everyone is called upon to do their part, taking every measure necessary to safeguard their own health and that of others.

Lightning Source UK Ltd.
Milton Keynes UK
UKHW022150211220
375642UK00009B/198